Joint Pain

by Kimmy Gerred

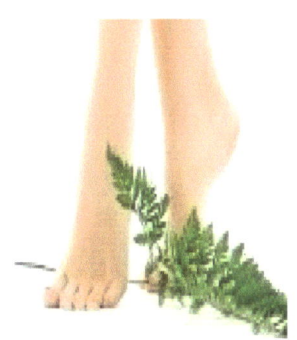

©Copyright 2017 Nelson Publishing Solutions

All Rights Reserved Copyright © 2017

By Nelson Publishing Solutions All rights reserved. This book or any portion thereof may not be reproduced or used in any manner whatsoever without the express written permission of the publisher except for the use of brief quotations in a book review.

Printed in the United States of America First Printing, February 4, 2017

Nelson Publishing Solutions   392 E. Stevens Rd. G13

Palm Springs, CA. 92262

- Pain has been found to be a precursor for heart disease
- Often inflammation causes pain
- Inflammation is a precursor to cancer
- Inflammation is just one of the many symptoms of joint pain
- Degenerative disease often causes joint pain
- Degenerative Disease can also be categorized as a form or type of arthritis

We hope to help you find natural and easy remedies to reduce or eliminate your joint pain and pain caused by inflammation.

This book is a personal home health care guide so we have left some blank pages for you to journal personal notes on or on each page for you to write in your own preferences or other tips that help you or your family members.

Use it like a living health journal of recipes and remedies for your family's home health care.

In this edition of "Joint Pain" we recommend that you drink lots of water, keep a daily food journal and eat lots of green leafy vegetables.

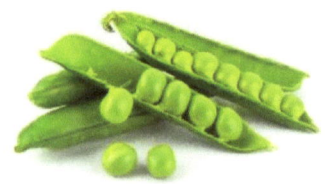

Drink lots of teas (especially green) and use lots of spices in your foods. And if you like ginger and cinnamon then you may even try both of them in your tea. It is a good idea to stay away from red meats, prepackaged foods, sugars, sweets (unless sweetened with a healthy substitute) and eat an apple a day too.

"Joint Pain" is a compilation of over 16 years of my personal self-study and University level studies.

As new information from new research presents new data and new statistics we will continue to update our readers on the latest treatments and discoveries.

All Vitamin and Supplement doses are to be taken as the label on the brand of your choice of purchase recommends unless otherwise stated by your doctor. Dosages for specific illnesses of cancer or arthritis are to be taken as suggested in this book unless your doctor tells you otherwise.

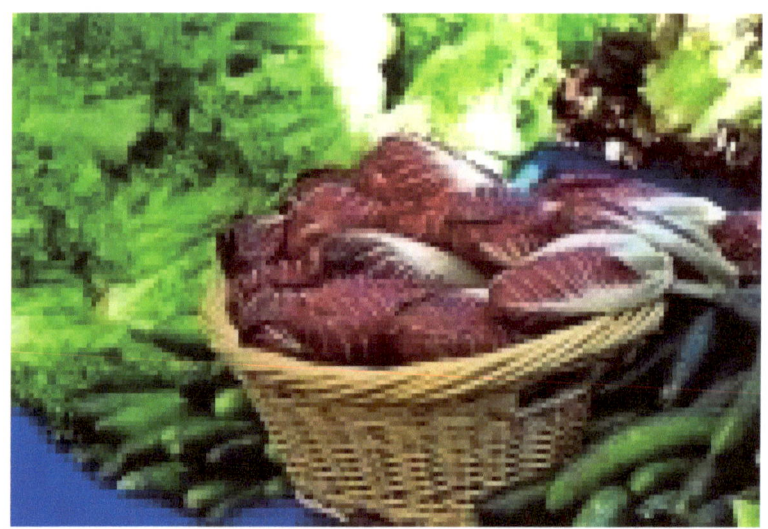

Prone to Arthritis?

Neutralize the pain within sixty seconds by rubbing **"Castor Oil"** directly into the affected area. Also, you can counter balance the effects of Arthritis with some foods high in these nutrients:

Coral Calcium

Vitamin E

Glucosamine and Chondroitin

Vitamin C

Vitamin A

Vitamin D

Juniper Berries

Boswellia

[Medical Marijuana, Hemp Oil Extract or high levels of CBD oil](#)

Or get it here http://tinyurl.com/MedMariJane

Ginger

Turmeric

Black Strap Molasses

MSM Collagen

Alfalfa Hyralonic Acid

Gelatin

You can also try this anti-inflammatory "[Defense](#)"

Here is the link:

[http://www.lnk123.com/aff_c?offer_id=614&aff_id=193678](#) for those reading the paperback version. Or try "[Eazol](#)" or "[Joint Advance](#)"

DAIRY

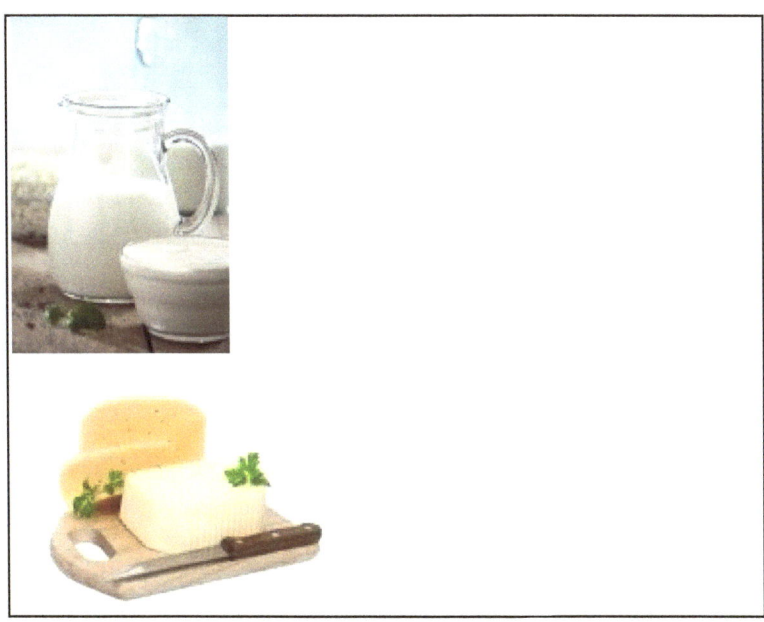

Dairy is a natural form of calcium. Although now they are saying that the phosphorus in the milk depletes the body of calcium and that we are better off getting our calcium from vegetables rich in calcium.

Try avoiding grains that cause inflammation. Inflammation is the cause of the pain in most cases. Bromelain Enzyme can be found naturally in Pineapples. Bromelain is an anti-inflammatory that really works fast on knee pain.

GINGER

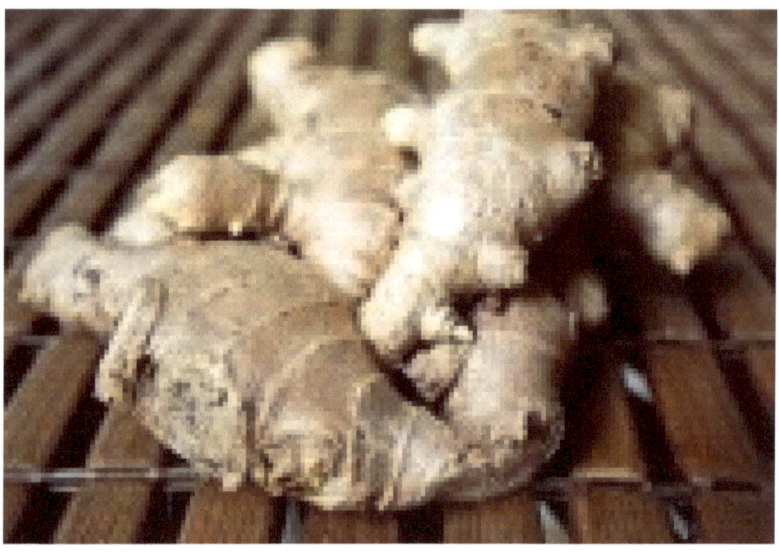

Ginger is another great for an anti-inflammatory.

Try to keep your body at a Ph of around 6 for optimal pain relief. Be aware of which foods trigger your pain.

Chemotherapy Treatment Success Enhancers:

Ginger greatly decreases nausea in Chemo patients. Selenium before, during and after Chemo greatly increases the success rate of healing as well as greatly decreases the chances of the return of cancer.

Gamma Vitamin E fights breast and prostate tumors.

Turmeric shrinks tumors

IP6

Black Strap Molasses turns blood alkaline which greatly reduces the chances of cancer. Find most of the vitamins here "[Health Buy Store](.)".

1 eight-ounce glass of water with ½ teaspoon of baking soda around 3PM each day.

1 eight-ounce glass of water with 1 teaspoon of apple cider vinegar each morning upon awaking.

Garlic cleanses the cholesterol out of the blood stream.

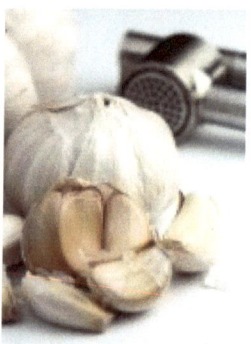

Dissolve Bone Spurs:

Acidic Calcium infused with K2

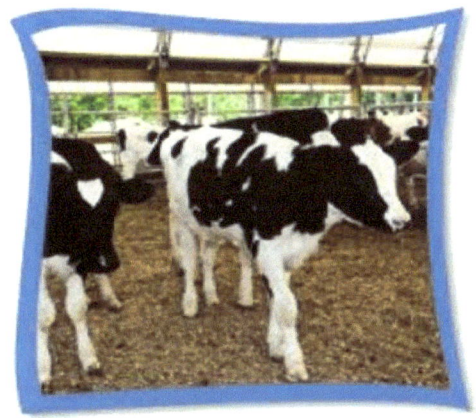

Find it here "[Health Buy Store]("

Chelation Therapy (Remove toxins build up):

Advanced Artery Solution

Saline Colonics

Colloidal Silver

Angio Prime

Omega 3

Lecithin

Garlic

COQ10

Vitamins D, E, & K,

Pomegranate Juice. (Compliments of Dr. Hans Petermann)

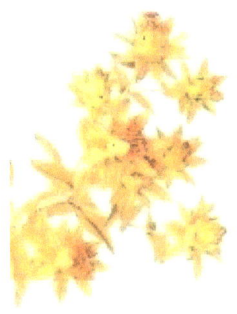

Appetite and Weight Control: Chromium Picolinate fights certain types of diabetes. [Acai Berry](#)

Tonalin CLA (Safflower Oil is where some CLA comes from) reduces belly fat in women rich in [anti-oxidants](#)

Green Tea helps curb appetite, [burn calories](#) and full of cancer fighting nutrients.

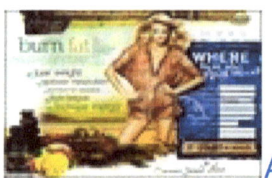African Mango reduces belly fat. And Drugs.com says "Research on African mango shows beneficial effects for diabetes and obesity, as well as analgesic, antimicrobial, antioxidant" www.Drugs.com

Alpha Lipoic Acid fights against neuropathy

Vinegar helps cleans the body of yeast

Kelp helps fight against virus' when combined with B Complex

Ginseng for added energy and stress relief

Aloe Vera Gel great for constipation and for enzymatic therapy.

Konjac fiber that makes you feel full Push away from the table a little take a walk or swim 30 minutes a day.

Hoodia Gardenia greatly suppresses the appetite.

Green Tea Weight Loss Program(Click Image To Order)

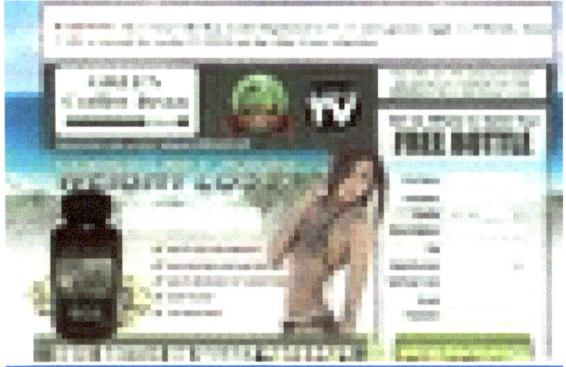

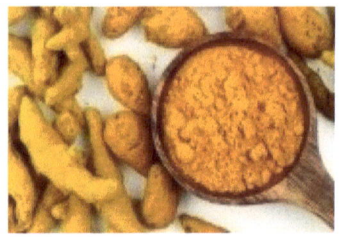

Prostrate or Breast Cancer:

IP6

Gamma Vitamin E 400IU

Selenium

Turmeric

Black Strap Molasses

Schizandra

3 cups of Green tea per day decreases breast cancer by 50%.

2 aspirin per week reduces risk of breast cancer by 20%

Vitamin D decreases risk of breast cancer by 20%.

Anti-Inflammatory "Defense"

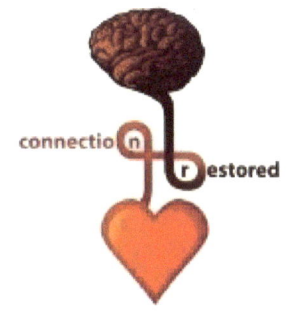

Recently it was reported that Pro football players are at greater risk of early Alzheimer's disease because of the multiple blows to their head. Obese African American women have greater risks and show symptoms of Alzheimer's much earlier than the other study groups. There are some wonderful natural ways to combat memory loss and stimulate brain health.

Brain Health:

Cumin and black pepper are good to detoxify brain tissue.

HGH

You can sprinkle turmeric on your eggs, along with sage, marjoram, basil, and garlic instead of salt.

Alzheimer's:

Ginkgo Biloba

Resveratrol

Pregnenolone

Vinpocetine

Coffee

Olive oil & Flax seed Oil

Cod Liver Oil

DHEA

Lecithin

L-Tyrosine

Rhodiola

Ashwagandha

Ginseng

Dl-Phenylalanine

Brain Health Continued on next page…….

Phosphatidylserine

Cumin

Black Pepper

[5HTP](#)

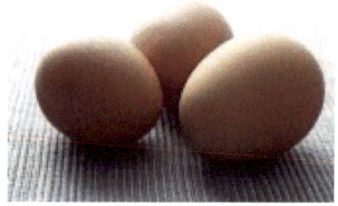

Lecithin is naturally found in eggs.

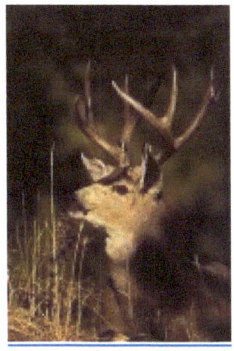

Erectile dysfunction or Impotence:

Ginseng

Deer Antler

Cayenne Pepper

L Arginine

Many drugs that are prescribed for depression will cause a loss of libido. Make sure that there is no strife between you and your spouse. Don't wander outside of your marriage and keep your priority on a good relationship.

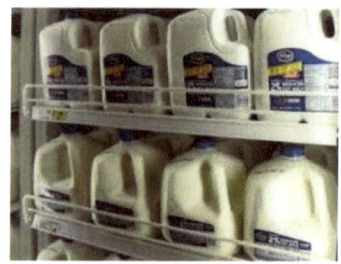

Bone Loss:

Coral Calcium

Collagen

Magnesium

Glucosamine and Chondroitin

Boswellia

Vitamin C

Vitamin D 3

Vitamin A

Vitamin E

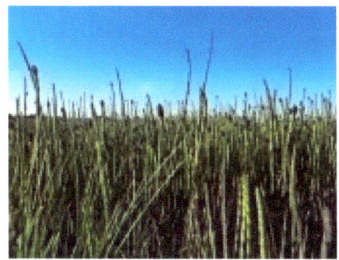

Cartilage Loss

Glucosamine and Chondroitin

Collagen

Cats Claw

Horse Tail Herb

Vitamin E

Vitamin C

Calcium

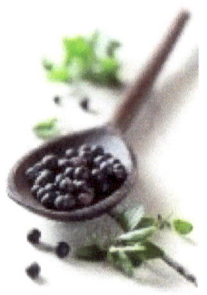

Fibromyalgia:

Juniper Berries

Black Strap Molasses

Ginger is great for digestion and reduces inflammation.

Turmeric shrinks tumors and fights inflammation.

Milk thistle detoxifies the liver.

Alfalfa turns blood level back to alkaline to reduce arthritic pain)

Pineapple Bromelain to detoxify, digestive aid and an anti-inflammatory that works great on knee pain!

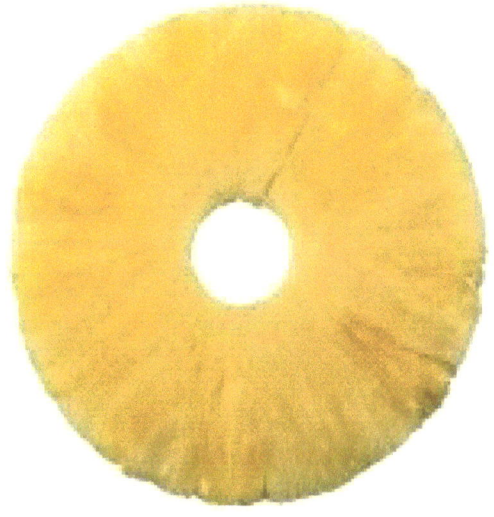

Tenninitis:

Cats Claw

Alfalfa

Black Strap Molasses (turns blood level back to alkaline reduce arthritic pain)

Ginger

Pineapple or Bromelain (will detoxify and act as an all-natural anti-inflammatory)

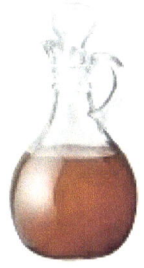

Chronic Fatigue:

B-Complex and Kelp

Plain Yogurt

Apple Cider Vinegar

Acidophiles (detoxify and anti-inflammatory)

Pro Biotics

Phosphatidylserine stops release of cortisol and helps with depression. Rest! A Stress free environment until complete health and wellbeing are restored for as long as necessary (depends on how chronic} It could take up to ten years in extreme cases where the immune system has shut down. Medical Science has proven that stress causes cancer. They have been teaching that in Modern Psychology since the early nineties. And they are still teaching it today in Social Science and Social Behavior Classes as I was a student of Psychology Holmes Community College Ridgeland, MS. In the early nineties and once again in 2011 I took another class on May 16, 2011 – "Stressed to the Nines: The Hard Truth about Anxiety and You "

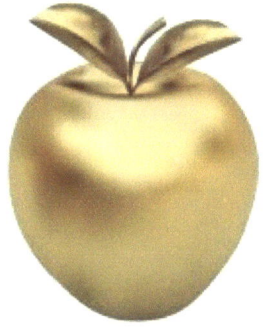

Constipation:

Cascara Sagrada

Senna

Wormwood parasite cleanser

Black Walnut Hull parasite cleanser

Slippery Elm

Old World Botanicals is a great place to find most everything mentioned in this book.

Esophagitis, Indigestion or Heart Burn:

Orange peel stops acid indigestion much faster and better than prescription ulcer medicine without the harmful side effects.

Licorice use like a sweetener in tea as a sugar substitute.

Bromelain

Aloe Vera gel

Apple Pectin or the skin of an apple.

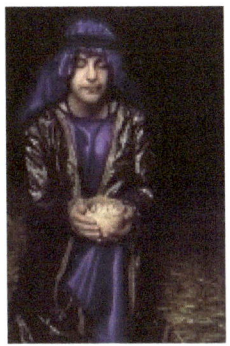

Pain Management & Anti Inflammatory:

Medical Marijuana, Hemp Oil Extract or high levels of CBD oil

Get it here: http://tinyurl.com/MedMariJane

Castor Oil (rubbed directly on the affected area)

Avoid Grains or any foods that trigger inflammation

Ginger

Turmeric

Boswellia

Black Strap Molasses

Fish Oil or Omega Fats

Bromelain

Alfalfa

Anti-Inflammatory "Defense"

Yeast Detoxification:

Plain Yogurt on empty stomach

Apple Cider Vinegar

Pau D' Arco

Pro Biotics Oregano oil

Caprylic Acid

Beta Glucan

Here is another great place to get answers for

Curing Yeast http://kimig.tripod.com/yeastcures/

Parasite Cleansing:

Crushed Papaya seeds

Black Walnut Hull

Cilantro

Garlic

Worm wood

Earl Grey

Bergamot tea

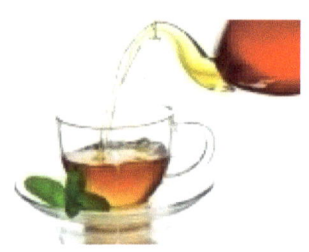

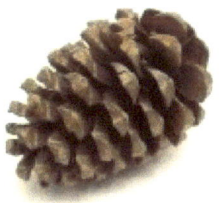

Hair loss:

Collagen

Horse Tail

B-Complex

Vitamin E

Pine Bark

Exfoliate scalp with honey, sugar and conditioner; apply in circular motion let sit for fifteen minutes then wash as normal.

Immune Deficiency:

Vitamin C

Selenium

Zinc

Colloidal Silver

Copper

Vitamin B Complex

Kelp

Vitamin E

Beta Glucan

DMG Mushrooms:

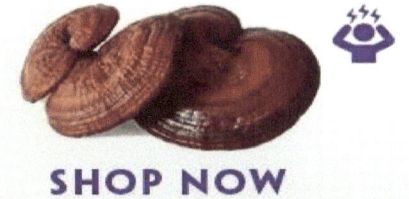

Maitake, Shiitake, Reishi,

Human Growth Hormone

Blue Berries

Grapeseed Extract

Manganese

Acai Berry

Dark Chocolate

Coffee

Co Q 10

Type 2 Diabetes control:

Garcinia Cambogia

Hoodia Gardenia

Gynostemma or Jiaogulan

African Mango

Chromium picolinate

Pine Nut

Tonalin CLA

Acai Berry

Green Tea

Alpha Lipoic Acid

Apple Cider Vinegar

Kelp B Complex

Ginseng

Aloe Vera Gel

Konjac (fiber that makes you feel full) Push away from the table a little take ride on a bike, a walk or swim 30 minutes a day.

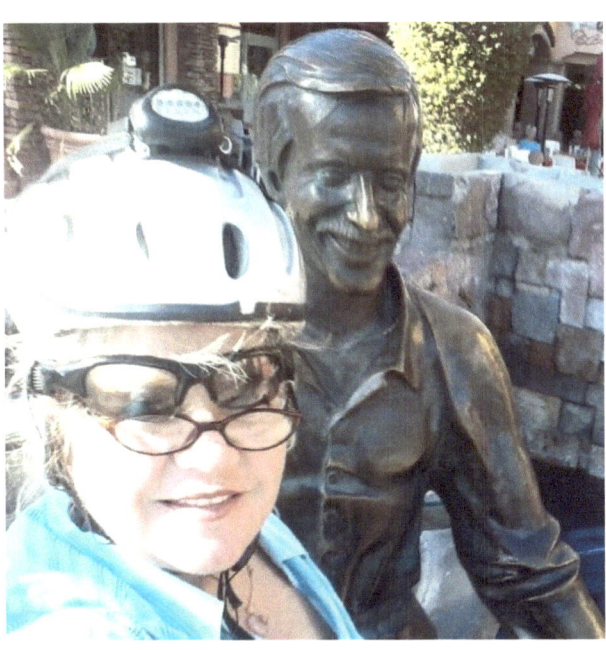

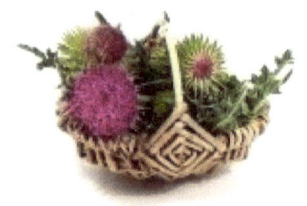

Hepatitis or other liver disease:

Milk Thistle

Burdock Root

Hyssop Red Clover

Green Vegetables

Echinacea

Insomnia:

Collagen

Dong Qui

Valerian Root

Magnesium

Melatonin (naturally found in Milk, Turkey, or Chicken)

Melatonin

Stay away from caffeine after 12:pm noon, avoid herbs like Ginseng, Guarana, and Guta Kola after 11AM.

Wrinkle Reduction:

Natural Alpha Hydroxy ie apple juice, sugar, or honey & brown sugar applied to the wrinkles at bedtime.

Remove with Corn meal facial scrub in the morning. Use plain coconut oil to moisturize.

Dark Circle Removal :

1. drop of Sweet Orange combined with 5 drops of grape seed oil
2. Witch Hazel (also helps with swelling)
3. Shepherds Purse (dissolve in water then apply)

To reduce swelling around the eyes:

Use 1/2 teaspoon of Preparation H cream only (not the oily ointment) and be sure not to get it near or in the eye. Apply to effected area.

To help heal the blood vessels around the eye use 2 Arnica tablets dissolved in 1 tablespoon of water apply one drop under effected eye.

Anxiety:

Lavender tea

Skullcap tea

Valerian Root

Magnesium

Dong Qui (take when needed or during ministration)

Phosphatidylserine (stops the release of cortisol)

Himalayan lamp (but you must not have it by the bed because the brain remains active around a Himalayan lamp)

Blood Clots, Restless Leg Syndrome or Varicose Veins:

Horse Chestnut

Aspirin

Vinegar rub downs

Ginger

Garlic

Onions

Niacin

Fever Few

Schizandra

Shepherds purse

Butchers broom

Lumbrokinase (Chinese Earthworm enzyme that eats blood clots it is also great for allergies)

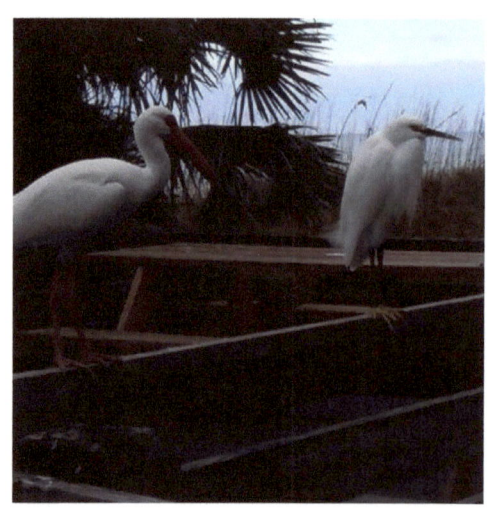

Poor Circulation:

Horse Chestnut

Schizandra

Aspirin

Hawthorne Berry

Fever Few

Niacin

[Cardiovascular](#) body movements.

Recently medical statistics revealed that people with poor circulation are at higher risk for heart disease and stroke. It is very serious and most heart tests do not reveal any problems in people with poor circulation when they are experiencing chest pain.

Be sure and see a medical doctor if you have chest pain. Butchers broom and Horse chestnut combined with Hawthorne Berry and Aspirin are more than enough to take the pain and inflammation away.

However, Hawthorne Berry is a very potent blood thinner and you must ask your doctor before taking it. You cannot take Hawthorn Berry prior to having any surgical procedures.

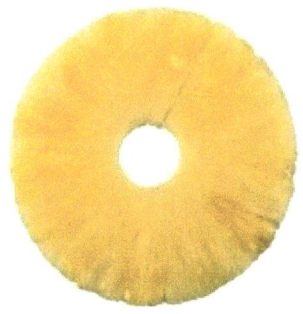

Inflammation:

Ginger

Turmeric

Boswellia

Black Strap Molasses

Willow Bark or better known as Aspirin Bromelain

or better known as Pineapple

Anti-Inflammatory "Defense"

Fish Oil (Recent studies have linked inflammation to heart disease and cancer)

(Click image to order anti-inflammatory "Defense")

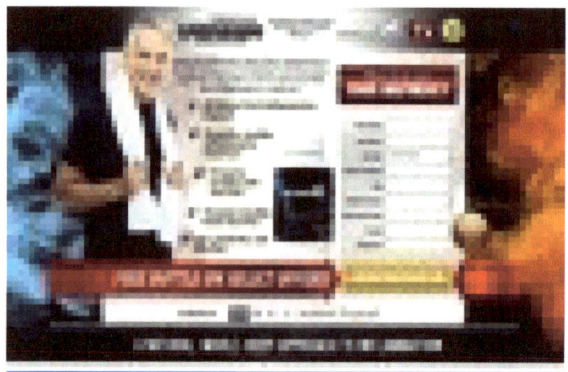

Sinusitis:

Xylitol nasal wash

Mullein

Olive leaf

Saline nasal wash (1 Quart of (distilled) water only, 2 tablespoons of canning salt 1 tablespoon of baking soda warmed to room temperature)

Bromelain

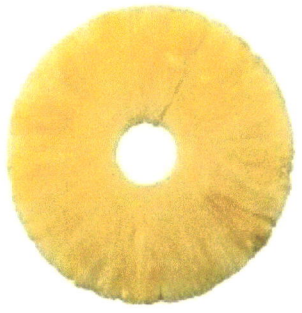

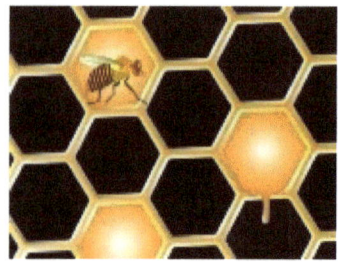

Allergies:

Bromelain

Mug wort

Bee Propolis

Mullein

Lumbrokinase (Chinese Earthworm enzyme that eats blood clots)

Cholesterol Control:

Garlic

Ex. Virgin Olive oil

Niacin

Polycosanol

Remove all butter and vegetable oil from your food. Replace butter with Extra Virgin Olive oil for a spread on your toast or potatoes. And you can also use the olive oil in your salad dressings.

Switch to Coconut oil to cook all your food with. This will eliminate bad cholesterol and help build up good cholesterol.

Heart Health:

CO Q10

Niacin

Garlic Fish Oil

Hawthorn Berry

Ribose

Horse Chestnut

Magnesium

Calcium

Ecotrin coated Aspirin

Polycosanol

Lumbrokinase (Chinese Earthworm enzyme that eats arterial blood clots)

Recently medical statistics revealed that people with poor circulation are at higher risk for heart disease and stroke. It is very serious and most heart tests do not reveal any problems in people with poor circulation when they are experiencing chest pain.

Be sure and see a medical doctor if you have chest pain. Butchers broom and Horse chestnut combined with Hawthorne Berry and Aspirin are more than enough to get rid of pain.

Anti-Clotting:

Ginger

Garlic

Onions

Shepherds purse or soldier's tea.

Feverfew

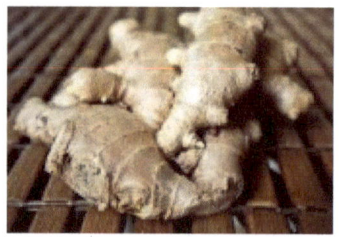

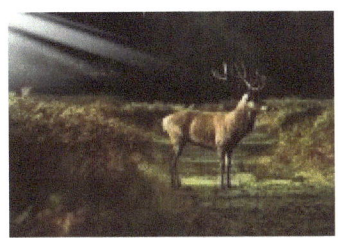

Deer velvet antler Has been scientifically proven to provide the following benefits:

Combating Cancer

Improving the Immune System Functions

Improving Athletic Performance

Stamina and Strength

Improving Muscle Recovery from muscle stress after exercise.

Also, an excellent natural supplement for Women's Health.

Providing Vitality and Anti-aging properties for Seniors.

Can be used as an alternative natural supplement for Bodybuilding and Weight Training.

Has an excellent source of Growth Factors including IGF-1 & IGF-2.

Improves and enhances sexual functioning for both men and women.

It's a natural supplement for Arthritis.

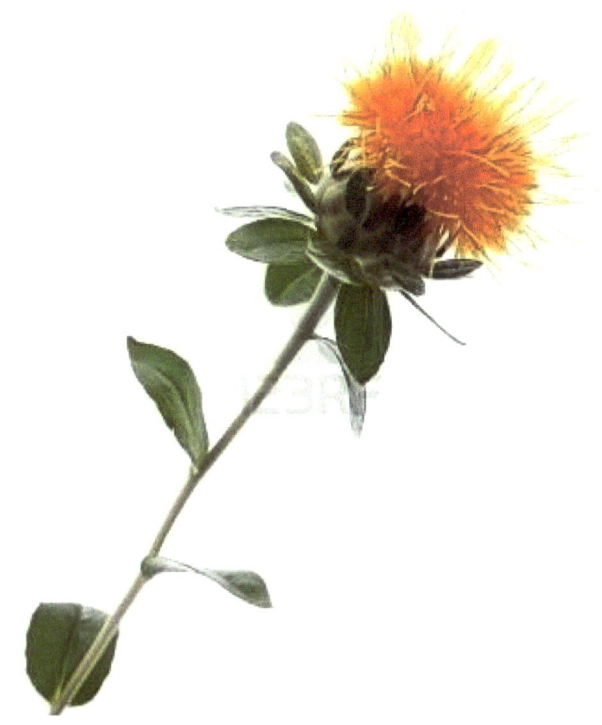

Relieve Depression:

Phosphatidylserine

[5 HTP](#)

St. John's Wart

Turmeric

Dill

Marjoram

Saffron

Nutmeg

Peppermint

Everyone benefits in health and in weight control when they switch ALL butters, vegetable oils, or fat back grease and replace all of those with Olive oil on toast, popcorn, salads, and switch to coconut oil for cooking.

You must not cook olive oil at high temperatures because it causes chemical structure to mutate and instead of being healthy it becomes a health hazard. On the other hand, Coconut oil can be cooked at high temperatures and it is very healthy just as olive oils are.

You will also find that there are many sugar substitutes such as honey or Xylitol that is much better for your immune system and the Xylitol will help fight cavities while trimming your waist. It looks and feels exactly like sugar does.

Recently Medical Research has discovered that Chronic Inflammation greatly increased the risk for women in stroke and heart attacks or heart disease. There is a new simple test to determine how much inflammation is in your blood.

See your physician to see if that is something that you need now. There are simple anti-inflammatory herbs and remedies mentioned above.

You can also start your day out with pineapple for breakfast. The enzymes in the pineapple help to breakdown the protein cells in the walls of cancer formation.

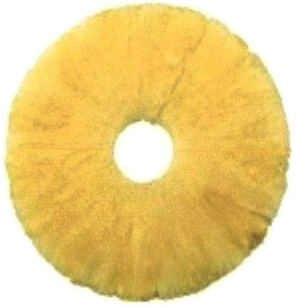

These are just a few simple ways that we have seen to bring great improvement for health naturally after years of research.

We use homeopathic remedies, herbs, teas, and supplements. We believe that the best cure is from the Great physician and creator the Great God Jehovah.

And that He has given herbs and nutrients that help us to maintain health by obeying His word and taking care of our temples (bodies) by respecting them with good health care practices.

One thing we all need each day of our lives is health!

Many are over stressed in over drive and have taxed the immune system to the point that it is shutting down.

In some cases, their bodies have excreted so much adrenaline from the Adrenalin Gland till there is not anymore "fight or flight" Epinephrine

[Epinephrine - Epinephrine (also referred to as adrenaline;) is a hormone and neurotransmitter. It is a catecholamine, a sympathomimetic monoamine extracted from the amino acids: phenylalanine and tyrosine. (Referring to the adrenal gland, which sits atop the kidneys and secretes epinephrine) When this happens our body becomes vulnerable to disease.

This will keep causing the body to continual release cortisol. It will wear down the immune system. Cortisol is what causes women to have too much stored fat in the belly. And maybe related to the rise in heart disease in women. In some cases, it is nearly impossible to stop this downward spiral of destruction because the chemical has such a profound effect on our brains that in turn effects our entire lives. But even the worst-case scenario can find hope in providing the body what it must have to function properly.

Let us help you to regain control of your health! Using all natural and botanical herbs combined with common sense, daily supplements of vitamins, minerals, and a healthy diet are basics that get the body back on track to optimal health. Rest is essential for the healing properties to manifest speedily. And a healthy environment is also important to get optimal results. We use a Healing Approach to master Disease Control and operate in Preventive Health care as well as Traditional and

Conventional Medicine applied conservatively. The Bible tells us that we are to obey our physicians and we would never counsel against your own doctors' advice. Most of our remedies can be found the kitchen cabinets anywhere, U.S.A.

And if there is a concern about a specific herb we would ask that you consult with your physician. Our goal is to help you feel better, look better, and live longer! We only provide Natural and Homeopathic Remedies. And for the most part, our goal of optimal health is obtained best by Preventive Health Care.

Natural Remedies are generally less expensive than prescription drugs, less side effects, and usually have more benefits than just healing a specific disease. For instance, the treatment for fighting cancer also fights inflammation.

These herbs in and of itself is not the cure. But combined with a healthy lifestyle pleasing to God and eating properly, that healing will be activated. There are some foods that must be abstained from and other foods that need to be partook of. It is like if you were eating foods with high calories and no vitamin or nutritional value, we need you to now do just the opposite, high vitamin, and nutritional value with very few calories. Spices and Teas are very beneficial in the healing process. In the Consultation, we can determine which ones are best for you.

www.ingramcontent.com/pod-product-compliance
Lightning Source LLC
Chambersburg PA
CBHW041105180526
45172CB00001B/119